Crystals for Healing

by Georgina Cyr

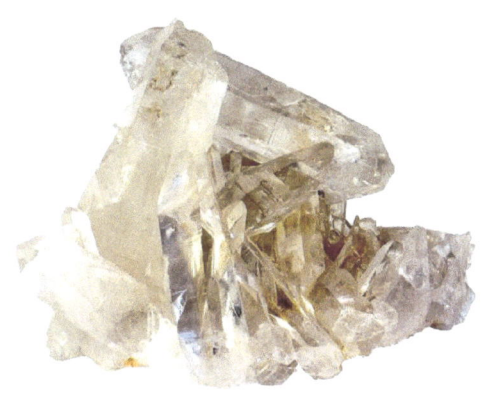

Georginacyr.com

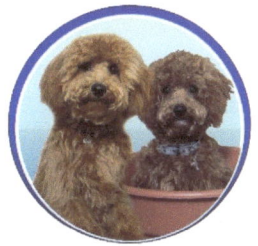

Table of Contents

History of the use of Gemstones for Healing

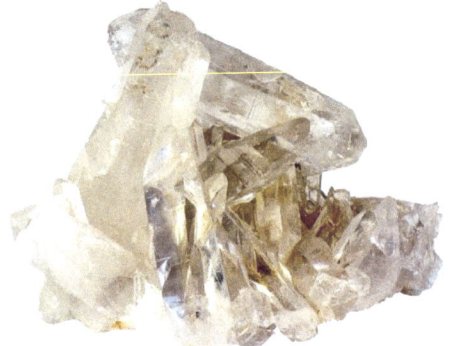

Archaeological research has shown that people have always collected gemstones. From the beginning of mankind, humans have felt the power of these gifts of the Earth. Records from the most ancient civilizations have shown that rocks, stones and gem formations have been used as talismans for good luck, admired for their beauty or form, and for the energetic healing they bring. There is evidence of the mining of stones, gemstones and crystals in Egypt over 7,000 years ago.

There are hundreds of references to the power of gemstones in the Bible. Exodus 28: 9-26 tells of the stones being chosen according to the names of the sons of Israel, for the breastplate of Israel's high priest.

In Revelation 21: 14 we read that the wall of the city had 12 foundation stones with the 12 names of the 12 apostles. Revelation 21: 19-20 tells the name of the stones that the foundation was made of. I think that from the beginning of time, all beings have been instinctively aware of the healing properties of stones.

Paracelsus was one of the first to research the healing properties of stones. Many cultures have used gems and stones as healing therapies. Historically the Vedas have contained the most extensive knowledge in the uses of gems and stones for healing. Some of the Vedas, such as Jyotish and the Guruda Purana described their use for physical, emotional and spiritual healing. Many of the treatments were done by creating liquid "essences" from the stones.

Kings and Queens wore stones and crystals for their "occult" powers, more than for showing personal wealth. The word "gem" itself refers to something of an exquisite or superior nature. Gems were used by Kings, Shamans, Witches, Wizards, Medicine Men and others to enhance health and spiritual wellbeing, and also manifest control and desire.

Crystals in Science
Crystals have both pieroelectricity and piezoelectricity.

Pyroelectricity

Pyroelectricity is the electrical potential created in certain materials when they are heated. As a result of a change in temperature, positive and negative charges move to opposite ends through migration, and hence an electrical potential is established.

Pyroelectricity can be visualized as one side of a triangle, where each corner represents energy states in the crystal: kinetic, electrical and thermal energy. The side between electrical and thermal corners represents the pyroelectric effect and produces no kinetic energy. The side between kinetic and electrical corners represents the piezoelectric effect and produces no heat. The first reference to the pyroelectric effect is in writings by Theophrastus in 314 BC, who noted that tourmaline becomes charged when heated. It will first attract ashes, and then will repel ashes, due to the electrical charges that change when heated.

Piezoelectricity

Piezoelectricity is the ability of certain crystals to generate a voltage in response to applied mechanical stress. The first practical application for piezoelectric devices was sonar, first developed during World War I. Intense development interest in piezoelectric devices occurred after the use of piezoelectricity in sonar and the success of that project. Over the next few decades, new piezoelectric materials and new applications for those materials were explored and developed. One of the best known applications is the butane fire starter, where a spring loaded hammer hits a piezoelectric crystal to ignite the gas over a spark jump. One of the other many things piezoelectricity can produce is electricity and light. *Note: This information was taken from the wikipedia free encyclopaedia. Please see the following web pages for more information.*
http://en.wikipedia.org/wiki/Pyroelectricity
http://en.wikipedia.org/wiki/Piezoelectric_effect#Mechanism

The Mohs Scale Classifies the Hardness of Stones

In 1812, the German mineralogist Frederich Mohs devised this scale that classifies the stones from the softest to the hardest.

Talc—easily scratched by the fingernail

Gypsum—just scratched by the fingernail

Calcite—scratches and is scratched by a copper coin

Fluorite—not scratched by a copper coin and does not scratch glass

Apatite—just scratches glass and is easily scratched by a knife

Orthoclase— easily scratches glass and is just scratched by a file

Quartz—not scratched by a file

Topaz - scratches quartz easily much harder than common substances

Corundum - scratches topaz and compares with the manufactured product called carborundum, though it is very different chemically. Sapphire and ruby are varieties of corundum. It is twice as hard as topaz.

Diamond - scratches topaz and corundum easily; is the hardest substance known. It is four times as hard as corundum.

How Gems work with the Physical Body

The composition of each gem, as nature created it, carries an energetic frequency, or wavelength. When gems are worn, they actually create an electromagnetic field around the person, animal or being. Each electromagnetic field will of course vary slightly in reaction to the vibrational frequency of the being using the gem.

The energy of the being using or wearing the gem transforms to create the changes necessary to promote physical, spiritual, and emotional well being.

Care must be taken to ensure you are using the correct stone for what you are looking to manifest.

The vibrations and colors of gemstones correspond to the vibrations and colors of the planets in our solar system. They also contain the life force of the earth. Each type of stone or gem has a unique vibration that can assist in releasing blockages of particular vibrations in our own bodies and help to facilitate our body's own ability to heal, as well as work with all energies and the more ethereal realms.

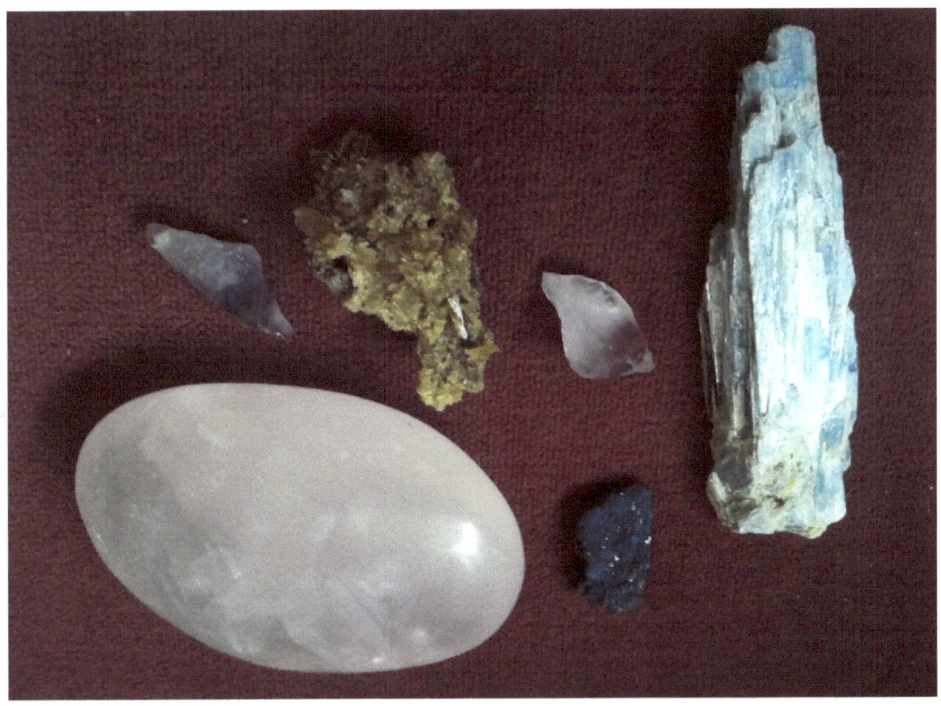

Techniques for using Crystals and Gemstones

When you begin to do any kind of work with energies or crystals, you need to be aware of your own energy.

Any emotional turmoil you carry inside of yourself will be picked up by the crystals, it it is always good to clear them before doing work on another being.

It is important to be in your space, balanced, centered, grounded, and have intentions of allowing the white light to work through you for the highest good.

When you work on any being, be connected to them so that you can really feel and sense their reactions to what you are doing.

Be prepared to go very slowly or to only work from a few minutes to an hour.

When the being is relaxing and sighing, or moving into you for what you are doing, you know that they are enjoying the session. Be very sensitive to their needs.

Remember your own energy and emotions and how you feel. Clear your own energy with white light, and be gently in your space before you start. Know that whatever crystals you choose to use, their energy will be amplified by your energy and your intent.

You need to be sure the crystal is appropriate and the energy of the crystal is appropriate.

You can also hold the crystal or stone in your hand and tune into your higher self to know how to use the crystal over the body.

You can gently move the crystal in the air over their body clockwise or in figure 8 movements.

Be very aware of the beings energies and try to tune into them to receive instructions from them or their higher selves.

You can lay them directly and gently on the being's body. Be sure to warm the crystals in your hands or in the sun first if you are laying them directly on the beings skin.

You can also put the crystal directly in the drinking water. Just be sure that the being will not accidentally or purposely ingest the crystals.

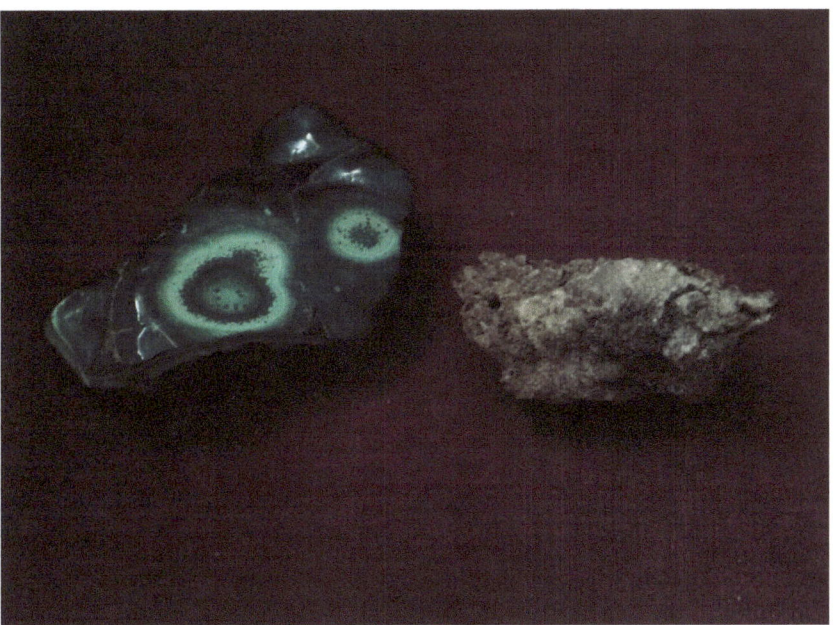

Clearing your Crystals

When do I need to clear my Crystals?

Crystals need to be cleaned whenever someone else handles them or works with them or when you use them to work with other people's energies.

It really depends how often you are using them and for what purpose. Use your own intuition as far as clearing them right after someone else handles them or looks at them for a few minutes. Just consider the energy of the person looking at or handling them. If you are comfortable with that person's energy, then you may just want to wait until it is convenient to clear them the crystal than getting all panicky about needing to do that right away.

Crystals have their own vibrational frequency and energetic properties, but as they work with their surroundings, whether on humans, animals or areas, they also absorb and carry the energy of that which they are working with. When one acquires a new crystal, stone or gemstone, it is important to clear the energy that it is already being carried before you start using it to work with your energy or another being's energy to ensure that you are not affected by the energy that the crystal has previously absorbed.

There are a few crystals which are said to not carry energy, they clear themselves. Two of the "self-clearing" crystals are Kyanite and Citrine.

It is important to remember that it is your intention in clearing the crystals that accomplishes the task. As we know, the white light energy has the highest vibration, and will clear any energy upon request. However, as with any being that has its own energetic vibration, the crystal has a purpose in what it does, and it may still be trying to work with its previous "job." Therefore, it is a good idea to not only use your intent of using white light to clear the crystal, but to put your intention into action by physically doing something to clear it.

Crystals can be cleared in many ways. Some crystals are very fragile and can be damaged by certain cleansing methods.

Common Methods of Clearing Crystals

- Put the crystal in salt water from the ocean or you can use pure sea salt to soak it in for 24 hours. Use a non metallic container.
- Run the crystal under running water with the intent of the water also carrying white light to clear the crystal.
- Leave the crystal in the sun for 4 hours.
- Leave the crystal in the moonlight all night. This works especially best on a full moon.
- Put the crystal into a safe area of a running river or stream for several minutes.
- Bury them in sand for 24 hours. The sand also grounds them to the earth.

Programming Your Crystal

When you acquire a new crystal that you want to work with, you will want to cleanse it first, and then introduce it to your intent. Some people call this dedicating or programming the crystal.

First get to know the physical and energetic properties of the particular kind of crystal you have. Introduce yourself to your crystal...this can be aloud or telepathically, and let it know that you honour it for its qualities and abilities.

Then tell your crystal what it is that you would like it to work on with you. You can do affirmations with your crystal, or talk to it as a friend.

It is always a good idea to treat the crystal that you are working with as you would a beloved pet. Be friends with it. Don't forget to ask the crystal how it would like you to work with it. Meditate or go into your space with it and ask it what it would like to share with you or teach you.

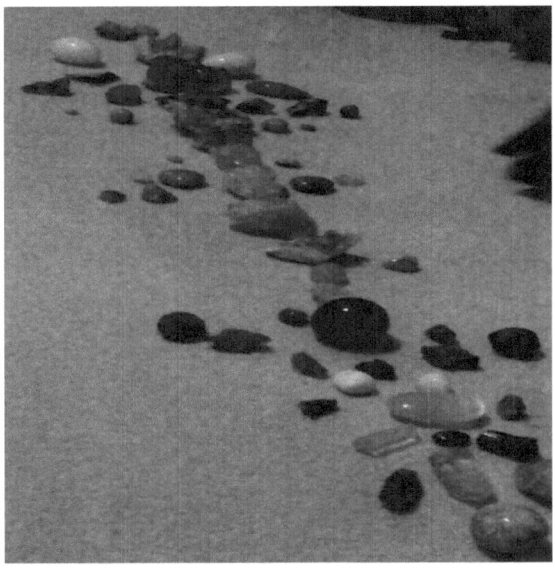

Common Crystals and Gemstones used for Energy Healing

Agate	Balances the yin & yang energies, assists in opening up intuition and telepathy. Helps to bring clarity, awareness and level thinking to a situation. Helpful for animals with lethargy or depression, only until a vet can diagnose the reasons behind them. Vibrates to the number 7. Astrological sign is Gemini.
Blue Lace Agate	Facilitates bringing in high vibrational energy for increased awareness and spiritual connectedness. Brings calming energy for animals having heated energy such as anger, short tempers and also helps heated physical conditions such as arthritis, by helping with circulation and moving energy. Vibrates to the number 5. Astrological sign Pisces.
Amber	Absorbs and clears negative energy, transmuting it into positive energy. Strengthens the immune system. Aids in healing by detoxifying and purifying the blood. Calming and soothing. Helps to manifesting needs and desires. Aligns physical and spiritual energies. Vibrates to the number 3. Astrological signs Leo & Aquarius.
Amethyst	Creates a feeling of peace and harmony for abused animals, eases separation anxiety, panic fear and grief. Transmutes lower energies into higher energies. Aids in healing the physical body and the emotional body. Helps with releasing unwanted outside energies. Works with animals that are over spirited or affected by outside influential energies, causing them to be stubborn or challenging of the alpha status. Restores self confidence after past abuse. Vibrates to the number 3. Astrological signs Pisces, Virgo, Aquarius and Capricorn.
Ametrine	Enhances consciousness and raises the spiritual vibration. Calms and soothes harsh energies replacing them with light and love. Releases negative blocks. Enhances harmony and compatibility in relationships. Helps to increase

	attention span for training, helps to calm and focus. Increases feelings of wellbeing, balances too much or too little physical energy…helps dogs that don't know when to stop even if they are tired. Vibrates to the number 4. Astrological sign Libra.
Apatite	Helps to balance over activity or under activity and to allow oneself to utilize information to think clearly for leadership or teaching roles. Helpful for animals in training for service to humans or other animals. Vibrates to the number 9. Astrological sign Gemini
Aquamarine	Gives confidence and courage. It is a stone of balancing spiritual energies and providing protection. Aligns the Chakras and the spiritual and ethereal bodies. Enhances connection to the higher self. Helps to calm and give compassionate tolerant energy. Helps for recovering from trauma. Vibrates to the number 1. Astrological signs Gemini, Pisces and Aries
Aventurine	Helps to heal the heart Chakra. Releases the memories that trigger fear and impulsive reactions to things that trigger those memories. Major abuse remedy for deep wounds. Good for any stress related to fear. Helps to calm when moving or doing stressful events like dog or horse shows. Helpful for flighty horses who are jittery ready to start and run at anything. Helps for confidence and enhances leadership qualities. Vibrates to the number 3 Astrological sign Aries.
Bloodstone	A healing stone and a stone of courage. Helpful in accepting change or re-alignment of energies. Enhances wisdom and harmony. Helps the body by working with the blood, liver kidneys and spleen. It is energy boosting for animals that are overcoming health challenges. It helps to release toxins from chemicals such as flea sprays or medical drugs antibiotics or pesticide chemical toxins. Good for heatstroke. Put the stone in water for overnight and give the water to the animal to drink. Vibrates to the numbers 4 and 6. Astrological sign Aries Pisces and Libra.

Boji 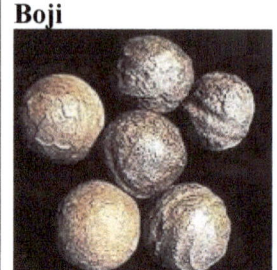	A stone created by a channeler in Colorado. It is blackish brownish and is primarily pyrite, has crystallization patterns and sometimes rainbows on the surface. Aligns the subtle bodies and the Chakras. It is really helpful in creating communication between species. It transfers energy from the etheric body to the physical body. It helps to strengthen the physical body and aids in healing. It enhances harmony and cooperation between animals and humans. Helps with training animals. A good grounding stone. Vibrates to the numbers 1 and 9. Astrological signs Aquarius, Scorpio, Leo and Taurus.
Calcite 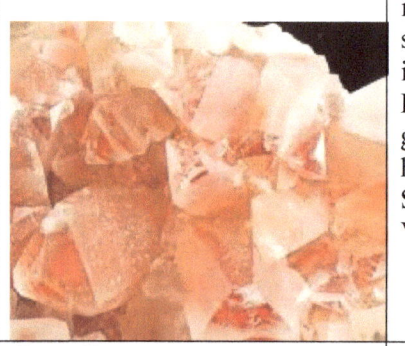	Is an energy amplifier. Helps one to remember information from one's higher self. Helps to access spiritual awareness and to integrate the astral information. Clears and activates all of the Chakras. Has been known to de-calcify the body of bone growths, increase circulation of energy and flow to help the body to heal. Orange calcite is helpful for S.A.D. for animals kept indoors with no sun. Vibrates to the number 8. Astrological sign – Cancer.
Carnelian 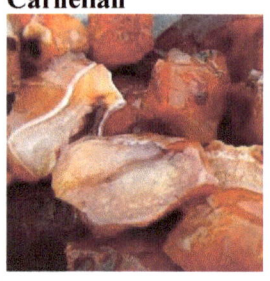	Enhances the love energy. Helps to increase the life force energy. Used for clearing unwanted energies and transmuting them to the light. Works to help mental abilities and concentration. Helps to release sorrow envy and fear. Helps animals to focus especially when day dreaming or seeming confused or not able to pay attention, great for training puppies. Vibrates to the numbers 5 and 6. Astrological sign Taurus, Cancer, and Leo.
Celestite 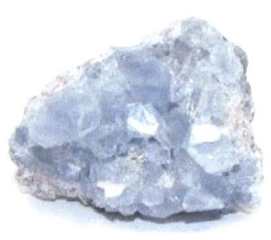	Helps with clarity of mind, helping one to understand how to integrate both spiritual information into ones life and help further ones development. It works with communication, delivering information from the Angelic realms. Assist in astral projection. Good for dream recall. Brings hope and faith in times of despair. Transmutes pain into loving light. Very healing. Vibrates to the numbers 2 and 8. Astrological sign – Gemini.

Chrysoberyl 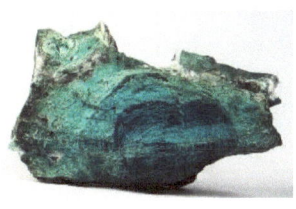	Helps one to attain perfection of personal power. Helps to release petty feelings and to move into a state of self worth and yet no ego. Allows one to understand all sides and the perfection in all things. Vibrates to the number 6. Astrological sign Leo.
Chrysocolla 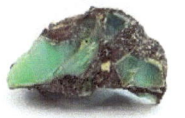	Helps to calm and give strength during stressful periods. Purifies the home and environment. Helps to release negativity from animals that have been abused. It allows one to open to the perfection of all, allowing peace and contentment. Helps to heal unresolved grief, trauma and stress. Vibrates to the number 5. Astrological sign Gemini, Virgo and Taurus.
Chrysoprase 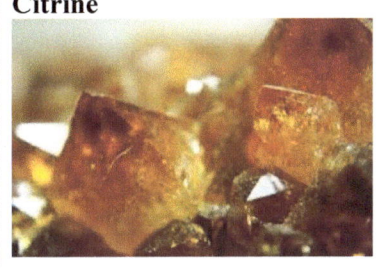	Opens the heart Chakra and aligns the Chakras with the ethereal realms. Helps to release the ego from superiority or inferiority complexes, allowing one to find the divine within. Opens up honesty and truth within oneself. Heals separation grief. Helpful for mothers who lose their young and are in mourning. Heals the heart of pain. Helps indoor animals to feel nature. Helpful for aggression. Vibrates to the number 3 Astrological sign Libra.
Citrine 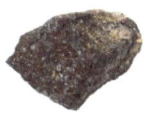	Dissipates negative energy, never needs cleansing. Attracts abundance & wealth and maintains it. It is good to place it in a cash drawer or wallet or purse for those reasons. Helps with pets who are moody fearful or awake during the night because of sensory overload. Works to dispel problems in the physical and energetic levels. Stimulates mental focus and endurance, good for training. Assists with solutions to problems. Helps to disperse fear and releases anger. Cleanses the aura. Vibrates to the number 6. Astrological signs Gemini Aries Libra & Leo.
Copper	Helpful for lethargy, apathy, restlessness and lack of focus. Stimulates optimism. Brings luck. Is a conductor of energy, helps transfer the energy from the source to the intended. Helps with circulation and has been known to help with arthritic conditions. Cleanses and purifies the system. Helps to ease fear of death. Vibrates to the number 1. Astrological sign Taurus & Sagittarius.

Emerald 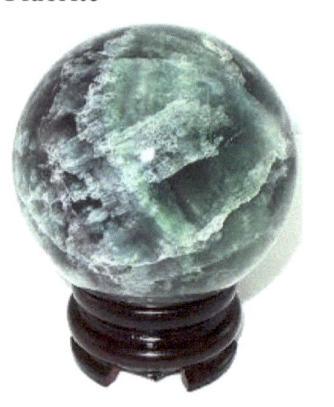	Facilitates sensitivity, love, bliss and harmony. Works with the heart Chakra. Eliminates negativity and brings forth positive. Helps with meditation. Helps with confidence in submissive animals. Calming and soothing. Astrological sign – Taurus, Gemini, and Aries.
Fluorite 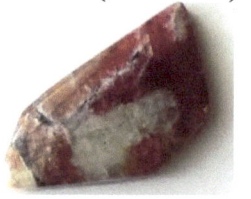	Calms disorganized chaos and confusion. A stone to enhance diplomacy. Increases ability to concentrate. Helps to promote harmony and peace in all situations. Helps to cleanse and assist health and harmony in the body, releasing blockages and stagnation. Helps with animals who feel scattered and distracted, helps them to comprehend and is said to raise the IQ. Vibrates to the number 7. Astrological sign Pisces & Capricorn.
Garnet- (Rhodolite) 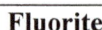	It extracts negative energy from the Chakras, and transmutes the energy into a beneficial state. Produces awareness and allows manifestation. Connects to the cosmic energies and stimulates the movement of the kundalini. Helps to allow for the perfection in All. Organizes disorganization. Works with the spine, heart lungs and blood. Helps to heal after surgery or trauma. Vibrates to the number 2. Astrological signs – Leo Virgo, Capricorn, and Aquarius.
Gold 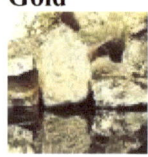	Acts as a healer for all body systems. Strengthens and regenerates the whole body, especially the nervous system protects against radiation and toxins. Helps with love and trust issues. Balances energy fields and allow release of inner conflict. Is the master healer. Works to purify the body. Vibrates to the number 2. Astrological sign Leo.
Hematite	Used for mental attunement memory enhancement and encourages optimism. Grounding and calming. Helps to stop panic. Works to strengthen blood

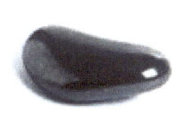	disorders contains iron. Also helps with kidneys Helps animal that have been abused and are showing signs of being worn down, who are physically depleted and have given up with no will to live. It helps restore their spirit as well as physical energy. Gives protection in negative environments. Vibrates to the number 9. Astrological sign Aries and Aquarius
Herkimer Diamonds– Quartz Crystals 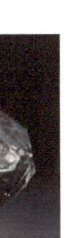	Good for communication clairvoyance telepathy. Astrological sign Sagittarius. Excellent stone for enhancing communication between species. It can retain information for later retrieval. Acts as a cleanser for the aura. Releases toxins and stress. Repairs ones energy field. It can be placed over areas of toxicity in the body to release the toxins and clear ones aura. Acts as an attunement stone to the environment or energy around one. Works to protect against radiation. Revitalizes spirit after loss of interest in life. Vibrates to the number 3. Astrological sign Sagittarius.
Jade 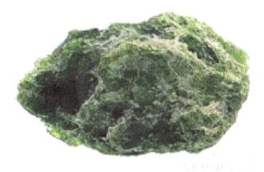	Helps with animals that have been recently rescued and are showing signs of fearful aggression. Helps calm stressed or anxious and reactive animals. Releases suppressed emotions. Transitions the spirit from the body to the spiritual world. Offers wisdom to problems. Opens one to love. Works with traumatic birth, and also skin and eye problems. Vibrates to the master number 11. Astrological signs Aries, Gemini, Taurus and Libra.
Jasper 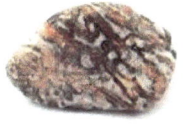	Helps in assisting others to discover themselves, nurtures contentment. Used for protection during travel. Used as a protection stone against negativity. Can align the Chakras and stabilize the aura. On a fast it can help to keep energy high. The ancients used it before astral travel for protection. It is a protection stone. It works with tissue degeneration of the internal organs. It is said to help balance mineral content of the body. Good for recovering aftershock or trauma. Good for indoor animals synchronizing earth cycles with the animals internal body rhythms. Vibrates to the number 6. Astrological sign Leo.

Kunzite 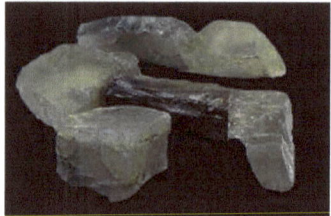	Activates the heart Chakra, bringing peace and purification on all levels. Opens one to the angelic realms. Helps remove obstacles form ones path, raises the vibration of the area around it. Dissolves negative energies, and dispels entity possessions. Produces a shield from unwanted energies. Good for meditation and assists one to be at peace in the midst of chaos. Can deflect radiation and microwaves from ones auric field. Vibrates to the number 7. Astrological signs – Scorpio, Taurus and Libra.
Kyanite 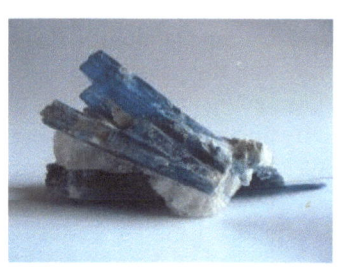	Helps for attunement – never needs cleansing – communication psychic abilities, meditation and dream recall. Used for aligning all Chakras, emotional intellectual, physical and spiritual bodies. It helps to release anger and brings a calmness and peace, to allow understanding and ability to reason. It facilitates awareness and enhances intuition. It is said to removes blockages in the body. Vibrates to the number 4. Astrological signs – Taurus, Libra, and Aries.
Lapis Lazuli 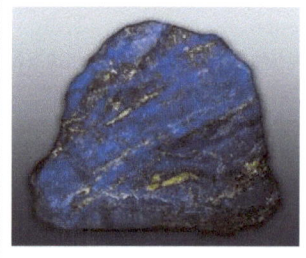	Connects one to sacred records of The All That Is. Helps to expand awareness. Helps to release ones baggage, useful for releasing past issues of abuse and pain. Helps to overcome depression. Enhances serenity in relationships. Helpful for guarding against physical attacks. Has been used to help disorders of the throat, helps with the immune system and is said to help hearing disorders. Vibrates to the number 3. Astrological sign Sagittarius.
Labradorite 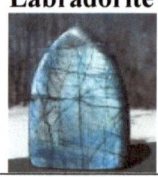	Helps with insecurities and releases disturbing thoughts. Helps one to let go of judgments, and allows one to just 'be". Vibrates to the numbers 6 and 7. Astrological signs Sagittarius, Scorpio, and Libra.
Larimar or Pectolite 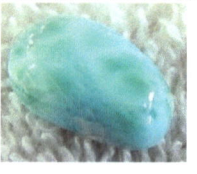	Helps to let go of guilt and allows forgiveness, stimulates deep understanding and serenity. Helps the spirit to release the feelings of bondage for animals that are kept indoors or contained. Larimar vibrates to the number 55 and Pectolite vibrates to the number 6. Astrological sign Leo.
Lazulite	Helps with addictions and compulsiveness. Calming.

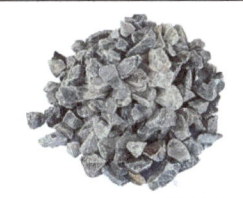	Excellent for anger hostility and frustration especially in horses. Vibrates to the number 7 Astrological sign Sagittarius and Gemini.
Malachite 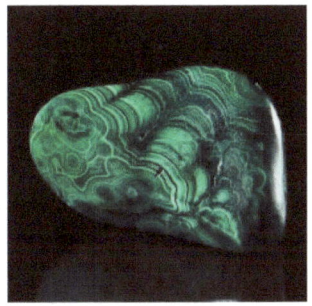	Helps with changes in life situations. Clears emotions and releases negative experiences that one cannot recall. Helps with weak body soul connections. Helps to protect against radiation and negative energies, whether physical or environmental. Assists in changing compulsive undesirable patterns in behaviour, mental confusion or disturbance. Helps with arthritic conditions, allergens, and motion sickness. Malachite has very high levels of copper and can lead to serious or fatal blood poisoning even if small amounts are swallowed. FOR EXTERNAL USE ONLY. Vibrates to the number 9. Astrological sign Capricorn and Scorpio.
Moonstone 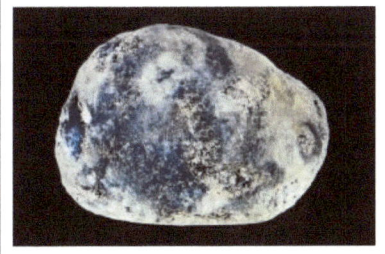	Brings harmony, peace, calmness and awareness in relationships. Soothes and relaxes stress. Helps with mood swings, balances hormonal stress and nervousness and emotions. Helps with changes and new beginnings. Helps to enhance feelings, insights and intuition. Used as good luck and protection for travelers. Said to help absorb nutrients and aid in digestion. Vibrates to the number 4. Astrological signs Cancer, Libra & Scorpio.
Onyx 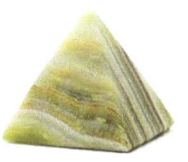	Helps to release grief, and gain personal strength, allowing happiness of the self. Vibrates to the number 6. Astrological sign Leo.
Peridot 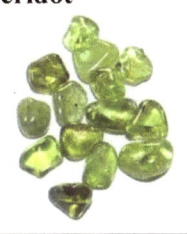	Eliminates toxins and helps with "life force" energy. Encourages peace and harmony, energy and vitality. Brings in the vital life force. Helps with adrenal glands. Helps to create harmony within the pack or human family and resolve jealousy issues, especially in cases of new family members. Helps with new anything - birth growth and changes. Vibrates to the numbers 5, 6 and 7. Astrological signs Virgo, Leo

	Scorpio, and Sagittarius.
Platinum	Balances the centers and meridians of the body. For animals that are intimidating or aggressively domineering, pushy or challenging regarding their placement in the pack. Animals who try to control their caregivers by becoming the alpha. Also helpful for depression creating aggression. Excellent for training. Helpful for eyes and digestion. Vibrates to the number 7. Astrological sign Leo.
Quartz	Receives stores, activates and transmits energy. It alleviates emotional extremes. Amplifies energy and thoughts for improved healing & immunity. Purifies the blood. Protects against radiation. Used in crystal massage to reduce pain and inflammation. Can be used to bring information from the Spiritual Realm. Helps with highly-strung or hysterical animals, helpful for a weak body soul link. Resonates with all Chakras. Known as the Master Healer. They contain the power to do anything. Vibrates to the number 4. Astrological sign of All.
Rose Quartz	Removes negativity. Helps with emotional healing. Eases resentment and hatred held from past abuse and feelings of being suspicious of new well meaning people. Helps for aggressive or hostile animals. It helps to open their heart Chakra allowing them to trust and love again. Gold would be good to use with Rose quartz in this instance. Vibrates to the number 7. Astrological signs – Libra & Taurus
Smokey Quartz	Has a calming and sedating effect and helps animals to adapt to changes in their environment, especially good for rescue cases, and helps with stress related diarrhoea. Good for calming and grounding during shock or trauma, such as an accident. Similar to a rescue remedy essence. Also Good for calming when an animal is to be worked on, for example us it before and during a horse has their teeth worked on. Also good for depression. Cleanses toxic energy from all aspects of the physical being. Helpful during travel. Vibrates to the numbers 2 and 8. Astrological signs Capricorn & Sagittarius.

Rhodochrosite	The stone of Love. Holds love energy and helps one to remain positive and full of dreams. Energizes and renews faith in life. Helpful in cases of denial or self negativity. Helps to bring light and love to aid in healing. Excellent for laying on of stones for healing the physical body. Vibrates to the number 4. Astrological signs Scorpio and Leo.
Rhodolite- Garnet	A type of Garnet. Helps healing of wounds, injuries, shock and trauma of the physical body. Repairs aura damage especially after injury or surgery. Move one from the state of dullness to the state of joy through inspiration. Helps with phantom limb pain, for example tail docking. Vibrates to the numbers 2 and 7. Astrological signs Leo, Virgo, Capricorn and Aquarius.
Ruby	Helps to protect against illness from a lowered immune system. Helps with confidence and brings joy back to the spirit after loss or grief. Helps with depression, apathy and poor concentration due to loss of a loved one. Amplifies energy, encouraging gentleness and dispelling violence. It lights the darkness. Vibrates to the number 3. Astrological signs Leo, Scorpio, Cancer and Sagittarius.
Selenite	Can be used to access past lives. Helps for diplomatic decision making and understanding. Helps to reduce free radicals in the body. Good for mental clarity and awareness. Good for the skeletal system and spine, and cellular structure. Can be used to access past and future lives. You can rinse it, but do not leave it in water as it will dissolve. Vibrates to the number 8. Astrological sign Taurus.
Sodalite	Calming, helps with creating group or family harmony, energy of fellowship, goals and purpose. Good for team sports. Work to bring a level of trust within the family or team members. Helps with logical thinking. Vibrates to the number 4. Astrological sign Sagittarius.

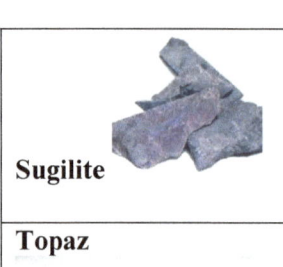 **Sugilite**	Helps to eliminate hostility and to bring one to a peace with being on this sometimes painful earth plane. Brings peace to the transition of death and dying. Vibrates to the numbers 2, 3 and 7. Astrological sign Virgo.
Topaz 	Helps with insecurities and doubts, allowing one to see the big picture and to not take everything so personally. Balances extreme emotions. Releases blocks from past trauma and pain. Has been used to correct disorders in the body. Vibrates to the number 6. Astrological sign Sagittarius.
Tourmaline 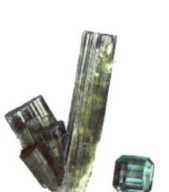	Works with the Chakras. Releases fear and encourages self confidence. Balances male and female energies. Provides insight in times of trouble. A shaman protection and dream, and helper stone. Helps to release the feeling of being a victim. Balances left and right brain. Vibrates to the number 2. Astrological sign Libra.
Black Tourmaline 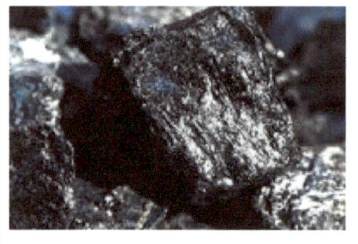	Protects against negativity. Revitalizes the victim and repels energy to sender. Protects against radiation. Brings vitality to the physical body, especially lower back. Helps animals who take on or absorb our energies. It helps to protect them from "our" stuff. Blocks radiation good for caged animals not allowed sunlight or nature; it can help with skeletal aches and pains and realign the bones and structural system. Vibrates to the numbers 3 and 4. Astrological Sign – Capricorn.
Turquoise 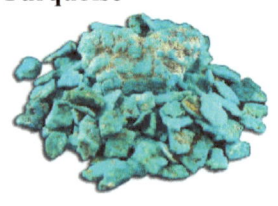	Master Healer – Used for Everything. Connects all, bringing the heaven and earth together in harmony with oneself. Can bring all energies to a higher level. Is a healer of the Spirit. Enhances wisdom and understanding. Used in Rain Dances. Good for grounding. Is a major stone for protection from all things real and unreal. Vibrates to the number 1. Astrological signs Sagittarius, Pisces and Scorpio.
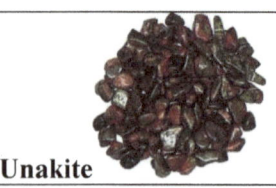 **Unakite**	Helps one deal with the past and assists in releasing the pain. Assists in weight gain in the areas desired. Vibrates to the number 9. Astrological sign. Scorpio.

Vogel Crystal	A quartz crystal cut in a triangular shape with smaller triangles on each side of the crystal to form a star tetrahedron or 6 pointed star when you look through it. It is the MerKaBa, the energetic "vehicle" that surrounds our bodies. Marcel Vogel designed this cut for healing and wore this type of pendant at all times when doing healing work.
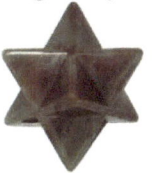	
Zoisite	Works to dispel negativity and transmutes the negativity to positive force fields. Has been called the fertility stone. Can be used to dispel laziness. Vibrates to the number 4. Astrological sign Gemini
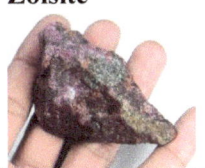	

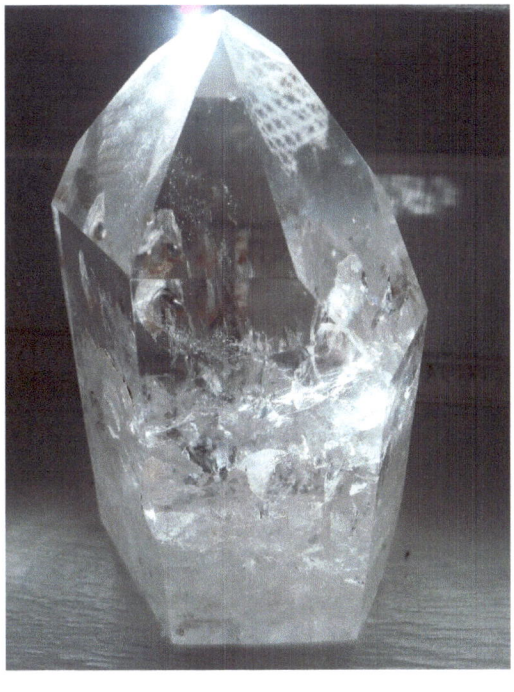

Crystal & Gem Practice Exercises

Exercise 1

Listen to a mediation CD or do a meditation on your own and connect with a crystal of your choice. Feel how it feels. Try to define the vibration of that particular crystal. Listen to what the crystal has to tell you. Take notes and follow the crystal's instructions as to how to use it. Pay attention to anything it tells you.

NOTES:

Exercise 2

Meditate with a Rose Quartz crystal. Feel its warmth and love. Ask it to show you the love in visual images... feel the love as you visualize it.

NOTES:

Exercise 3

Part A - Meditate with a piece of Carnelian. Ask it to share its properties and energetic frequency with you. Ask it for new knowledge.

NOTES:

Part B - Because its properties are for helping one to clear the mind and help the memory, carry it with you at a specific time when you need your clarity of mind enhanced for a specific purpose. After the exercise, record what you have experienced and how it has helped you.

NOTES:

Exercise 4

Meditate with a piece of Turquoise. As Turquoise is a master healer, ask it if it will share its many different abilities with you. Try to feel each property. Come out of the meditation just enough to write the properties down and then go back into the meditation to gather experience of another property. This exercise is good practice for going in and out of a meditation without losing the connection.

NOTES:

Exercise 5

Shamanic Journey Crystal…Going into a meditation, tune into a Kunzite crystal. Kunzite crystals are particularly good for giving information from the Shamanic or psychic realms. Ask for direction as to how to use the information from the experience.

NOTES:

Conclusion

There are numerous ways to incorporate the use of crystals into your life. I hope you will be able to use the information I have given you to create harmony and happiness into your life.

Thank you for giving me the opportunity to share this information with you.

Light Blessings,

Georgina Cyr

www.ingramcontent.com/pod-product-compliance
Lightning Source LLC
Chambersburg PA
CBHW050922290526

45792CB00002B/863